ECHINACEA

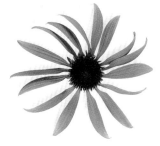

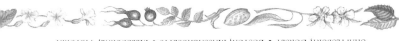

SHAFTESBURY, DORSET • BOSTON, MASSACHUSETTS • MELBOURNE, VICTORIA

ELEMENT

JILL ROSEMARY DAVIES

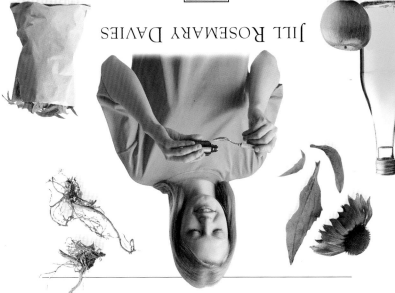

ECHINACEA ANGUSTIFOLIA
ECHINACEA PURPUREA

ECHINACEA

IN A NUTSHELL

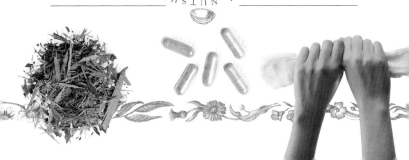

_ 9).
For growing and harvesting, calendar information applies only to the northern

NOTE FROM THE PUBLISHER

Any information given in this book is not intended to be taken as a replacement for medical advice. Any person with a condition requiring medical attention should consult a qualified practitioner or therapist.

Published in Australia in 1999 by
ELEMENT BOOKS LIMITED
and distributed by Penguin Australia Ltd
487 Maroondah Highway,
Ringwood, Victoria 3134

Published in the USA in 1999 by
ELEMENT BOOKS INC.
160 North Washington Street,
Boston MA 02114

First published in Great Britain in 1999 by
ELEMENT BOOKS LIMITED
Shaftesbury, Dorset SP7 8BP

© Element Books Limited 1999

Jill Rosemary Davies has asserted her right under the Copyright, Designs, and Patents Act, 1988, to be identified as Author of this work.

Designed and created for Element Books with
The Bridgewater Book Company Ltd.

ELEMENT BOOKS LIMITED
Managing Editor Miranda Spicer
Senior Commissioning Editor Caro Ness
Editor Kate John
Group Production Director Clare Armstrong
Production Manager Susan Sutterby

THE BRIDGEWATER BOOK COMPANY
Art Directors Emma Smith/Kevin Knight
Designer Jane Lanaway
Project Editor Lorraine Turner
Editorial Director Sophie Collins
DTP Designer Chris Lanaway
Picture Research Lynda Marshall
Photography Guy Ryecart
Illustrations Michael Courtney

Printed and bound in the UK by Butler and Tanner, Frome.

Library of Congress Cataloging in Publication data available

British Library Cataloguing in Publication data available

ISBN 1 86204 503 8

The publishers wish to thank the following for the use of pictures:
A–Z Botanical Collection: p.27b.
Bridgeman Art Library: pp.10r, British Museum, London; 12l, Reynolds Museum, North Carolina. Private Collection.
E.T. Archive: p.11r. Image Bank: pp.11b, 23, 45r. Garden Picture Library: pp.8, 10b. Science Photo Library: pp.18, 20r. Copyright © 1998 Steven Foster: pp.1, 9r, 27t. Stock Market: p.20b.

Special thanks go to:
The School of Herbal Medicine, Hailsham, West Sussex, UK

Contents

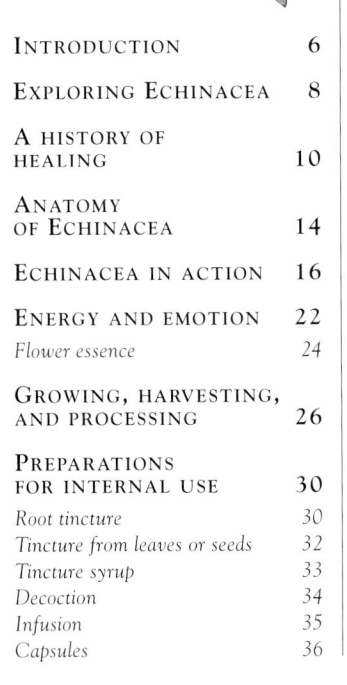

Introduction

THE SACRED PLANT of the Native Americans, Echinacea is considered to be the most beautiful of North American wild flowers. Common to the prairies, it is widely found in the eastern part of North America, from Canada to Texas.

The flowers resemble daisies

Echinacea is a sturdy-looking plant with branching stems and dark green leaves. It may grow to be 2–5ft (60–150cm) tall, depending on the soil and species. This perennial plant usually takes 2–3 years to produce flowers, which bloom in midsummer. The flowers, which look like large daisies, are 6in (15cm) across with petals arranged like rays around a central protruding cone. Seeds ripen in the fall, after which the plant dies back.

The head and petals can grow to 6in (15cm) in diameter

DEFINITION

Botanical family: *Compositae* (related to the sunflower family *Asteraceae*)
Species: There are eight species, but only three are significant for healing. *Echinacea angustifolia* and the larger *Echinacea purpurea* are the two species favored for commercial use, while *Echinacea pallida* is used to a small extent by those who harvest their own plants. *Echinacea pallida* is paler in color than the other two species, and its herbal effects are weaker.

RIGHT **Echinacea angustifolia, *one of the three species of Echinacea used by herbalists.***

Echinacea angustifolia *grows to about 2ft (60cm) high*

The dark green leaves grow at the base of the plant

THE HEALING SPECIES

Echinacea angustifolia is the commercial favorite. It has distinctive, narrow, lance-shaped leaves, and the flowers vary in color from pale pink through to pale or deep purple. It generally has a single tapering root.

ABOVE *Echinacea is both beautiful and rich in healing qualities.*

Echinacea purpurea is taller and stouter with larger, oval-shaped, coarsely toothed leaves. Its flowers are slightly longer and droopier than E. angustifolia, with reddish to dark purple petals. Its fibrous roots and rootlets can be found comparatively near the surface of the soil.

Echinacea pallida grows up to 4ft (120cm) in height. Between May and August it produces pale purple coneflowers up to 4in (10cm) long. As its name suggests, its effects, as well as its color, are weaker than those of E. angustifolia and E. purpurea, so this book will concentrate only on the two stronger species.

The Latin name Echinacea is derived from the Greek word echinos, meaning "sea urchin" or "hedgehog," and comes from the prickly appearance of the plant's seed head in the fall – and perhaps to some extent from the central coneflower in the summer. Angustifolia describes the plant's narrow leaves; purpurea describes its strong purple flowers; and pallida describes its pale flowers.

WHAT TO BUY

Use certified, organically produced Echinacea for the best healing potential. You can grow your own from seed, although it will be a couple of years before you will have seeds you can harvest; or you can purchase dried flowers and leaves, and whole or ground Echinacea root, from an accredited herbalist or herbal supplier (see page 59).

Exploring Echinacea

NATIVE TO NORTH AMERICA, *Echinacea species are lime-loving plants, which prefer well-drained but moisture-retentive soil. When seen in the wild, they create a wonderful vision of color.*

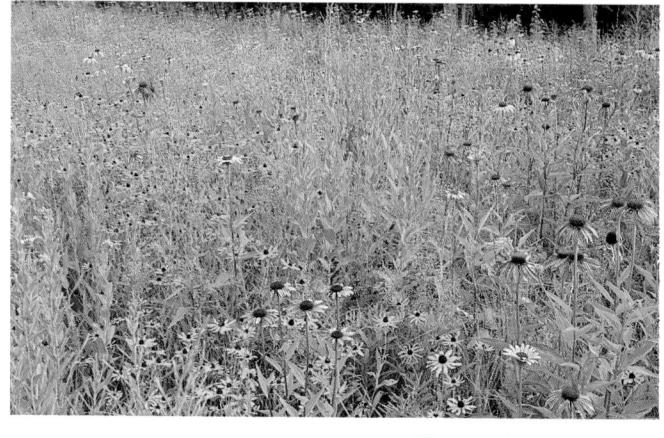

ABOVE **The purple flowers of Echinacea** purpurea **stand out in this meadow of wild flowers.**

WHERE TO FIND ECHINACEA

*E*chinacea angustifolia grows wild in the dry uplands and rocky plains of several American states, notably in Texas, Kansas, Colorado, and Montana. However, *E. purpurea* can be found more widely in eastern, midwestern, and southern states, particularly in the thickets and open woods of Virginia, Pennsylvania, Missouri, and Arkansas; it is also found in southern Canada. All Echinacea species are naturally tolerant of frost and drought – they are very hardy and adaptable.

COMMERCIAL GROWERS

Echinacea is commercially produced throughout the United States and New Zealand, and in British Columbia, Canada. The herb also grows in Europe, mainly in Germany and, to a small extent, in Britain.

SOIL REQUIREMENTS

Most species of Echinacea are lime-loving plants (6–8 pH) and grow best on fertile, free-draining, loamy or peaty soils. Although newly planted seedlings need frequent watering in the first month, this becomes less important later. In New Zealand, however, *E. purpurea* has produced better fields of crops when it has been grown in soil with a pH of 5.5–6. In Germany, growers consider that light, friable soils are best, since these soils can easily be washed off the roots when they are harvested commercially.

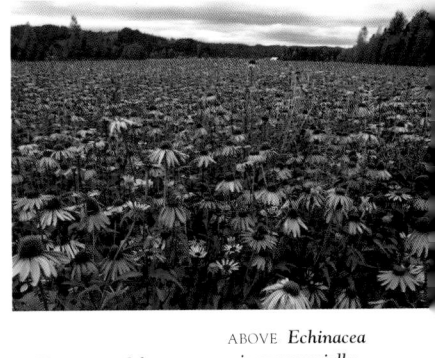

ABOVE **Echinacea is commercially cultivated in New Zealand.**

E. angustifolia yields are much higher under cultivation than in the wild, provided that the soil is well aerated and has balanced amounts of moisture, light, heat, and nutrients, but they perform poorly on continuously saturated soils. Echinacea will also thrive in dry clay loam if it is not allowed to become too wet; to prevent this, add gravel, sand, or fibrous compost.

BOVE **The roots of Echinacea lants like loamy or peaty soils.**

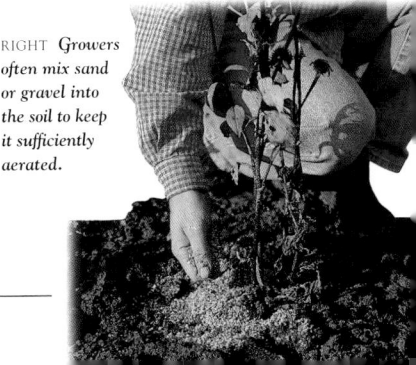

RIGHT **Growers often mix sand or gravel into the soil to keep it sufficiently aerated.**

A history of healing

NATIVE AMERICANS *often referred to Echinacea as a "sacred herb," but the names they would have used in their own dialects have been lost. The Plains Indians used Echinacea medicinally more than any other plant, and they may well have chosen names to reflect its "cure-all" status.*

Although its Native American names have not survived, Echinacea gained many common names when white settlers learned of its use about 200 years ago. These names provide insight into its appearance and its use in the past. **Purple Coneflower**, for instance, simply describes the species *E. purpurea*; **Missouri Snakeroot** reflects the plant's use to treat rattlesnake bites, as well as the fibrous appearance of

ABOVE **Echinacea purpurea,** *complete with roots and flowers.*

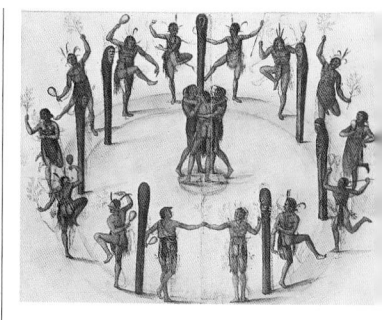

ABOVE *Native Americans used herbs in fertility rituals as well as in medicines.*

E. purpurea's roots; **Purple Kansas Cornflower** conveys one of the areas where this plant can be found growing wild; **Indian Head** recalls its use by Native Americans. Other common names include **Sampson Root, Black Sampson,** and **Red Sunflower**.

RIGHT *The name "Purple Coneflower" aptly describes the flowers of* E. purpurea.

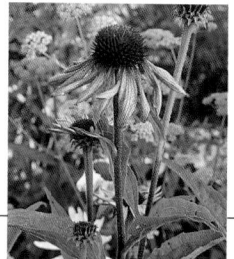

TRADITIONAL USES

Native Americans, especially the Plains Indians, used various species of Echinacea, both internally and externally, to treat a range of conditions. One of its main external applications was to treat poisonous insect bites and snakebites. They also used it for healing boils and all kinds of skin irritations, and to bathe burns and other external skin problems. It was taken internally for breaking fevers, for complaints such as sore throats, toothache, mumps, even headaches, and for major ailments such as smallpox and measles. They also added the juice to the water sprinkled on coals during traditional "sweats."

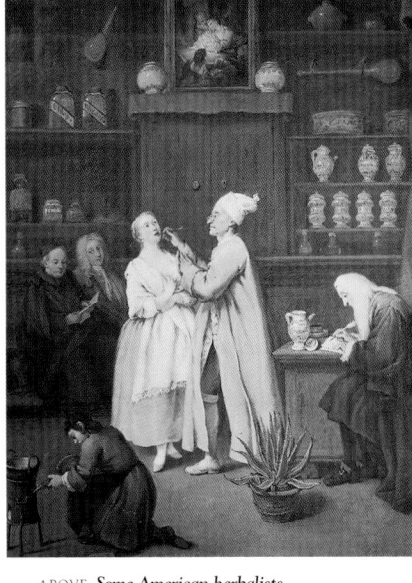

ABOVE *Some American herbalists in the 19th and early 20th centuries promoted Echinacea.*

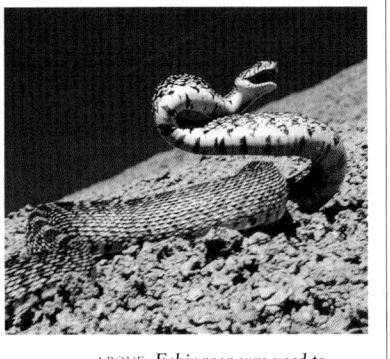

ABOVE *Echinacea was used to treat rattlesnake bites.*

HISTORICAL USAGE

A German physician named Dr. H. C. F. Meyer, who was living in Nebraska in the 1870s, formulated his own medicinal version of Echinacea and called it "Meyer's Blood Purifier." A champion of the plant's healing properties, Dr. Meyer typified the 19th and early 20th century interest in the herb, which derived from European interest in the uses to which Native Americans put it.

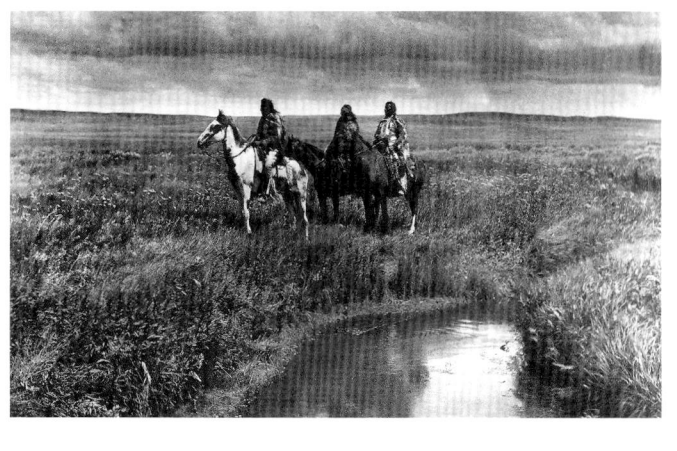

Today's natural healers recognize that the Native Americans had a very advanced system of healthcare based on sound natural healing methods. The Native Americans were renowned for their attention to nutrition and, of course, their use of herbs, in which Echinacea featured prominently. Their healing methods also included sweating and fasting.

The Cheyenne and Winnebago tribes have records verifying the widespread use of Echinacea across the nation, and archeological exploration of sites dating from the 17th century has produced evidence of its use for a variety of ailments.

ABOVE *Native American tribes held Echinacea in high esteem as a panacea for themselves and for their horses.*

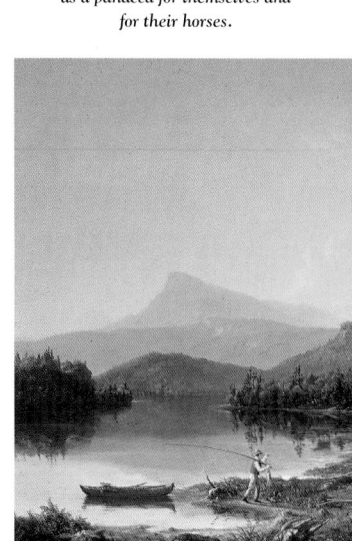

According to historical evidence, different tribes used this plant for different reasons: the Cheyenne used it to treat sore mouths and gums, the Dakota used it for bowel problems and tonsillitis, and the Delaware used it for gonorrhea.

White settlers gained their plant healing knowledge from the local tribes who lived around their settlements.

The Native Americans showed the white settlers how to use fresh Echinacea, picked in the summer, as a general infection fighter, and the settlers developed it as a tincture for winter use.

LEFT *A tincture preserves the herb's healing qualities.*

BELOW *Early white settlers in the Midwest learned the uses of Echinacea from the Native Americans.*

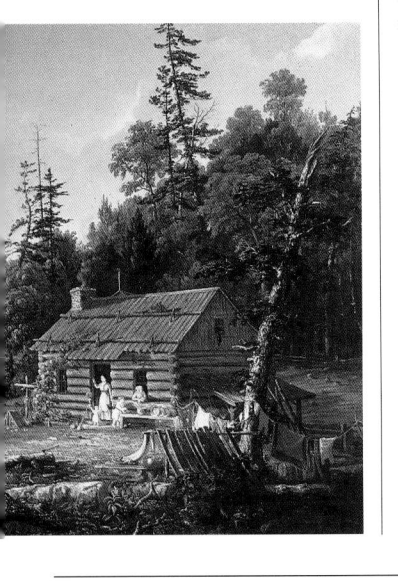

ECHINACEA IN WESTERN MEDICINE

Echinacea was brought to the forefront of Western herbal medicine by the Eclectics, a group of doctors who based their medicine on the use of herbs. The Eclectics came together in the early 19th century; they were prominent for a century from the 1830s. Schools of that era still survive in the United States and Europe. Echinacea also became more prominent under the auspices of a well-known Eclectic doctor and author called John King, who wrote the famous *King's American Dispensary*. Several American herb companies making tinctures from Echinacea were famous in their day. One such firm was Lloyd Brothers.

ECHINACEA LEAVES

Anatomy of Echinacea

THE WHOLE ECHINACEA PLANT *can be used for therapeutic purposes. Different parts are processed and preserved in different ways, depending on the use.* Echinacea angustifolia *is the most commonly grown and manufactured species.*

ABOVE **The fibrous roots of** Echinacea purpurea.

ROOTS

Echinacea angustifolia has a vertical taproot, whereas *Echinacea purpurea* has branched, fibrous roots and rootlets.

Chemical constituents
Polysaccharides, including inulin, a water-soluble carbohydrate; phenolic compounds: caffeoylechinacoside and cynarin; many alkylamides, including echinacein; essential oils such as caryophyllenene and humulene; alkaloids: tussilogin and isotussilagin, plus behenic acid; carbohydrates: sucrose, pentosans, and fructose.

SHELF LIFE OF ROOTS
dried, cut, or shredded root lasts up to 1 year; dried whole root lasts for 1–2 years.

STEMS AND LEAVES

The stems and leaves of *E. angustifolia* are covered with coarse hairs. The leaves are stalked, but become stalkless and smaller toward the top of the plant. The leaves are prominently veined, with five veins running bladewise. *E. angustifolia* has dark green, oblong, lanceolate (lance-shaped) leaves (see page 6). The leaves of *E. purpurea* are more oval in shape and are rich green in color.

SHELF LIFE OF LEAVES
whole leaf lasts 6–12 months;
shredded leaf lasts 6–9 months.

Chemical constituents
Phenolic compounds:
verbascoside, caftaric acid,
chlorogenic and isochlorogenic
acids; flavonoids: luteolin,
quercetin, and rutoside; essential
oils: vanillin, germacrene D;
hydrocarbons, N alkanes,
betaine hydrochloride.

FLOWERS AND SEEDS

Echinacea angustifolia has
large, single, daisylike
flowers at the ends of stems or
branches. These flowers have
narrow, strap-shaped petals that
are indented with two or three
notches at the tips. The flowers
are quite short, and spread
rather than droop; their coloring
varies from rosy pink to pale
purple. The flowers have a
prominent seed-bearing "cone,"
which is browny orange with
scattered yellow pollen. The
seeds, which erupt from this
cone in the fall, are medium size
and brown in color.

Chemical constituents
Phenolic compound: chicoric
acid; numerous miscellaneous
alkylamides; essential oils,
including vanillin; considerable
amounts of vitamin C.

SHELF LIFE OF
FLOWERS AND SEEDS
flowers last 6–12 months;
seeds last 1–2 years, but they
will last much longer with
suitable storage facilities.

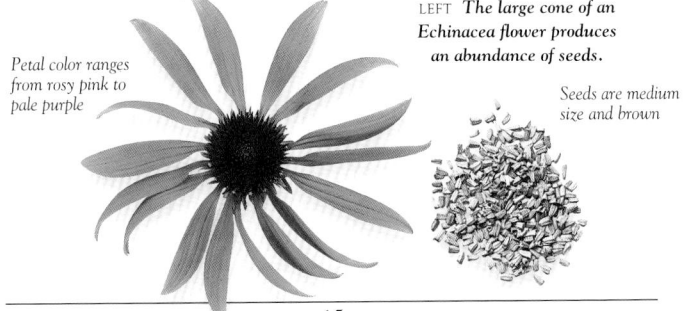

LEFT **The large cone of an**
Echinacea flower produces
an abundance of seeds.

Petal color ranges
from rosy pink to
pale purple

Seeds are medium
size and brown

Echinacea in action

THIS WONDERFUL, ALL-ROUND HERB *can be used to treat the young, the middle-aged, and the elderly alike. It is able to boost the immune system to fight many viral, bacterial, and fungal-based diseases, and is a known lymph cleanser and herbal antibiotic. There are not many conditions that this immune system stimulant cannot help.*

ABOVE *Taking Echinacea alleviates the symptoms of colds and flu.*

HOW ECHINACEA CAN HELP

❧ Ideal as a cold or flu aid, this herb can be taken when you first feel shivery, right through the illness, and for a week afterward in order to aid full recovery.

❧ Useful for coughs, and other more deep-seated or chronic bronchial and upper respiratory disorders, including asthma and whooping cough.

❧ Alleviates any signs of enlarged glands and lymph nodes, and any attendant sore throat or tonsillitis.

❧ Gives quick relief from food poisoning and eases the severity of the symptoms.

❧ Helps in the treatment of psoriasis, skin ulcers, boils, abscesses, eczema, infected wounds, bites, and burns, both by external

LEFT *Echinacea is particularly effective with coughs and other problems of the upper respiratory tract.*

application as an ointment and internal use.

❧ Useful in cases of candida and other fungal-based diseases.

❧ Helps in the treatment of urinary tract infections such as cystitis and urethritis.

❧ Helps to treat pelvic inflammatory disease and other infections of the female and male lower reproductive systems.

❧ Assists recovery from chronic diseases such as postviral fatigue syndrome (formerly known as ME), and may aid in recovery from some cancers (except where white blood cells are excessively produced or compromised in some way, for example, with leukemia and autoimmune diseases such as rheumatoid arthritis).

HOW ECHINACEA AFFECTS THE BODY

Echinacea should make the whole mouth tingle quite strongly and make it feel slightly numb. The effect starts quite gently, increases to the point where extra saliva is created, and then dies down after several minutes. This process suggests that Echinacea stimulates the immune tissue situated under the tongue. The initial effect will be stronger with E. angustifolia than with E. purpurea.

Echinacea will then make its way to the ileum of the stomach, where it stimulates the Peyer's patches (immune tissue). These patches in turn trigger "immune stations" located throughout the body, which creates all-round protection. Such immune stations include the bone marrow, where immune system cells are created, and all the lymph nodes and vessels that carry white blood cells and help to filter and purify the blood. The spleen will also be activated.

The whole mouth tingles and feels slightly numb

Echinacea seems to stimulate the immune system tissue under the tongue

Immune stations are triggered

RIGHT **The first effects of Echinacea are quite noticeable in the mouth.**

EFFECTS

❧ Continuously produces white blood cells in large amounts to help fight general infection.

❧ Creates large killer cells called macrophages or "big eaters" (see page 57), along with other types of immune system fighter cells.

❧ Stimulates the growth of new, healthy tissue.

❧ Protects cells from invasion or damage by pathogens, bacteria, or viruses.

❧ Increases the body's overall ability to dispose of bacteria, infected and damaged cells, toxins, and harmful chemicals.

❧ Stimulates the adrenal cortex, and produces an increased amount of cortisol. Cortisol is a steroid hormone that helps the metabolism of carbohydrates, aids the body's normal responses to stress, and eases inflammation and the accompanying pain.

> ### CAUTION
> Echinacea stimulates the body rather than supporting it. In fact, after prolonged use, it can cause the immune system to underproduce some disease-fighting elements. For this reason it should only be taken in short bursts or cycles, coupled with herbal tonics and good nutrition. You should also always keep to the recommended dosage.

SUMMARY

Echinacea helps to treat a wide variety of surface conditions effectively, as well as a range of deeper-seated diseases of the immune system. Surface conditions include those of a more superficial nature, such as a cold, where Echinacea's extra immune system helps speed recovery. In a deep-seated condition, such as postviral fatigue syndrome (ME), where immunity is compromised, the herb's ability to reactivate an immune system response can help the body to fight the spread of the disease. However, if the body's immune system is excessively depleted, Echinacea alone will not be able to reactivate it.

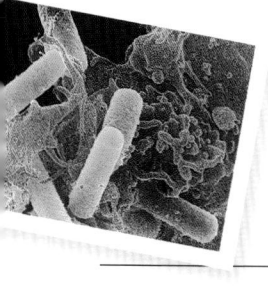

LEFT *Micrograph of macrophages, disease-fighting cells that defend the body.*

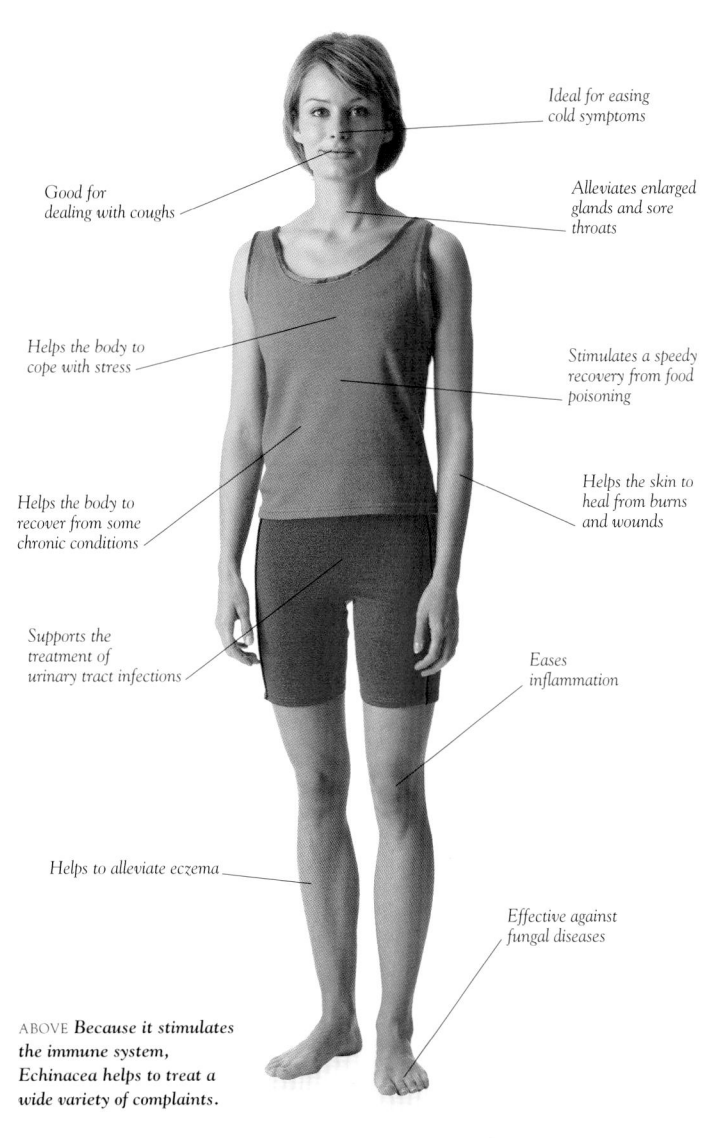

Ideal for easing
cold symptoms

Alleviates enlarged
glands and sore
throats

Good for
dealing with coughs

Helps the body to
cope with stress

Stimulates a speedy
recovery from food
poisoning

Helps the body to
recover from some
chronic conditions

Helps the skin to
heal from burns
and wounds

Supports the
treatment of
urinary tract infections

Eases
inflammation

Helps to alleviate eczema

Effective against
fungal diseases

ABOVE *Because it stimulates
the immune system,
Echinacea helps to treat a
wide variety of complaints.*

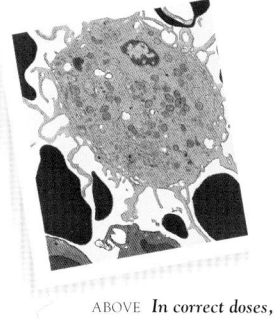

ABOVE **In correct doses,
Echinacea stimulates the body's
natural fighter cells that attack
and destroy invasive cells
and infections.**

PROVEN RESULTS

Some of Echinacea's healing properties have been tested scientifically and shown to work.

❊ Clinical studies of the use of Echinacea, undertaken in 1989, showed an increase of 50–120% in immune system function over a five-day period.

❊ Other studies, conducted with 4,500 patients who had inflammatory skin conditions (including psoriasis), showed that 85% of patients had their symptoms relieved with topical applications of Echinacea salve.

❊ Laboratory experiments in 1985 showed that white blood cells stimulated by Echinacea increased their infection-fighting activity. This led to an increase in the consumption of yeast cells by 20–40%, proving Echinacea's usefulness in the treatment of fungal infections such as candida (thrush).

WHEN TO AVOID ECHINACEA

Echinacea is generally a very safe herb and is well tolerated by most people of different ages and races. Currently, it is believed that no part of the plant is toxic. However, due to the broad and nonspecific nature of the way it stimulates the immune system, Echinacea should not be given to people with progressive systemic and autoimmune disorders such as lupus (SLE),

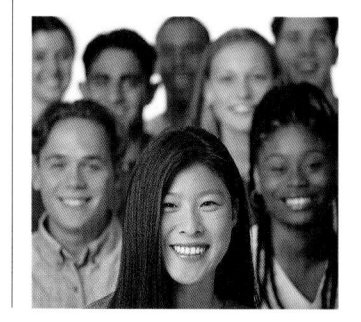

RIGHT **Echinacea seems to
work with people of all races
and ethnic backgrounds.**

collagenosis, and related disorders. It should also (according to the German Kommission E) not be used with tuberculosis. Other conditions for which Echinacea is not recommended are multiple sclerosis, rheumatoid arthritis, and leukemia.

Echinacea may also counteract some aspects of chemotherapy, where the chemotherapy is being given to suppress the function of the immune system. If you are having this type of chemotherapy, avoid Echinacea.

ALLERGIC REACTION TO ECHINACEA

In the spring of 1998, an allergy specialist warned that very occasionally people with allergies who take Echinacea at the same time as drinking fruit juice could trigger an allergic response, even anaphylactic shock. One of the people who sustained such an adverse reaction had been taking Echinacea for many years, on its own or with water. On just one occasion she put it in fruit juice and reacted immediately.

Anaphylactic shock is a serious, life-threatening emergency, and the sufferer must have an injection of adrenaline as soon as possible. If this happens to someone you know, call an ambulance or take the person to the nearest hospital emergency department immediately. An anaphylactic reaction to Echinacea may start with a burning in the mouth and throat, tightness in the chest, and diarrhea. The symptoms may stop at this point or proceed to more dangerous levels.

> **CAUTION**
>
> If you have kidney disease, restrict your use of Echinacea to 10 days at a time. This will help to avoid possible imbalances caused by the herb stimulating the production of too many salts and minerals.

LEFT *Anaphylactic shock is a life-threatening reaction that must be dealt with at once. It often starts with burning in the mouth and throat.*

Energy and emotion

GOOD QUALITY ECHINACEA *produces a tingling, numbing effect in the mouth, especially the species* E. angustifolia. *This has the effect of creating extra amounts of saliva, which in turn excites the production of digestive juices in the mouth and gut.*

According to traditional Chinese and Ayurvedic (ancient Indian) medicine, taste has its own part to play in contributing to the healing properties of a herb. Echinacea has a very

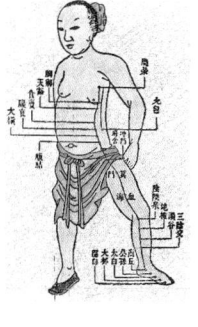

LEFT **Traditional Chinese medicine treats illnesses via body channels.**

metallic taste – similar to chewing metallic wrapping paper on an exposed tooth. Other underlying flavors are bitter, pungent, and slightly sweet.

According to traditional Chinese medicine, all of these flavors support the lungs, stomach, and liver, which in turn ultimately regulate the immune system.

In traditional Chinese and Ayurvedic medicine, the "metal" taste of Echinacea belongs to the season of the fall, and the organs affected are the lungs and large intestine. The large intestine (classed as male) and the lungs

HELPING DIGESTION

In addition to its other properties, Echinacea is also a digestive herb in its own right, partly due to its Betaine HCL (Hydrochloric acid levels). This helps the body to digest food more efficiently. It also lessens the likelihood of leaving undigested food, which can ferment and cause wind and acid indigestion. Echinacea can deal with excessive or harmful amounts of bacteria, fungi, and other unfriendly microorganisms, and their unpleasant side effects.

ABOVE *Echinacea's metallic taste has been ascribed to the fall.*

(classed as female) are seen as forming a partnership.

The lungs and large intestine are two areas of the body that have to stay clean and healthy in order for them to perform correctly; they represent the very basic functions of life – breathing and excreting.

ENERGY AND THE MIND

The taste of Echinacea is strong and stimulating, and can make the body feel empowered instantly. Creating extra saliva is generally a reassuring process: when we are frightened our mouths go dry, but producing extra saliva is relaxing and produces more endorphins (pain-relieving hormones). The result is that Echinacea will make you feel more capable or even pleasantly excited.

TRADITIONAL CHINESE MEDICINE

Traditional Chinese medicine evolved as a complete medical system over thousands of years, through practical method, observation, experience, and experiment. Coming from a civilization that perceives people as being either "in harmony" or "out of harmony" with themselves, traditional Chinese medicine sees illness or disease in terms of patterns of disharmony. Accordingly, what it tries to do is to restore the correct balance in the body of the sick person.

Practitioners believe that diseases are caused by an imbalance in the four elements within a person: wind, heat, dampness, or cold. The illnesses are treated via meridians, the channels in the body through which energy is believed to flow. Herbs used are classified according to four categories:

- Four Natures
- Five Flavors
- Four Directions
- Organs and Meridians affected by them.

RIGHT *Echinacea's distinctive taste can make the body immediately feel fitter and more active.*

FLOWER REMEDIES

Echinacea has the ability to lighten your mental load because it can lift from your shoulders anxieties about survival and immunity. You can relax, you don't need to be so self-protective, and you'll be able to welcome other things into your life. The shape of the flower is also important: it is very round and whole and the color is a strongly spiritual one – these features can help you to move to higher levels of change and consciousness.

Because Echinacea can give a feeling of empowerment, it can help you to welcome changes and new challenges. It is also protective and purifying.

Echinacea flower essence stimulates and awakens the true inner self, and this quality makes

TO MAKE A FLOWER ESSENCE

STANDARD QUANTITY

Approx 1½ cups (350ml) each of spring water and brandy, and 3–4 Echinacea flowers

1 *Carefully select some Echinacea flowers that look healthy and strong. Then choose a very quiet spot indoors – or in a secluded area of the yard or sunny woodland if the weather allows. Place the flowers, while still fresh, in a glass bowl with the spring water, ensuring there is enough water to cover them and that they are fully submerged.*

2 *Cover the bowl with clean white cheesecloth; put in a sunny position.*

RIGHT **Extracting Echinacea flower essence provides a stimulating restorative for body and soul.**

it a fundamental remedy for many physical conditions – and for those of the "soul."

The flower essence is especially good for those who have been shattered by severe trauma or abuse, such as bereavement, child abuse, long-term exhaustion, and lowered immunity, as well as a deep sense of rejection, loneliness, or lowered self-esteem.

3 *Leave the bowl in the sunshine for several hours – perhaps next to a window if you are indoors. Try to ensure that the flowers have at least three hours of continuous sunshine. If they wilt sooner than this – which they may do in fierce sun – then they can be removed earlier.*

4 *After the three hours or so remove the flowers and discard them, using a twig to lift them out of the bowl.*

5 *Add an amount of brandy equal to the remaining amount of water-and-flower mixture, to preserve the liquid. Pour the liquid into dark glass bottles and label carefully.*

PLANT SPIRIT ENERGIES

The spirit of the Echinacea plant is different from that of a flower essence, which is connected mostly with the flowering of the plant. The whole of the Echinacea plant is of benefit in healing – flowers, seeds, stem, leaves, and roots, so it is the whole spirit of the plant that enables each of these parts to share their energy with us.

Because it is so powerful, Echinacea is able to treat deep genetic tendencies that are part of an individual's constitution. It helps balance old patterns of behavior physically, mentally, and spiritually.

CASE STUDY

James had been diagnosed with infectious mononucleosis by his G.P. He was told that there was little that could be prescribed to make him feel better, and that he would be laid low for some time. His wife had read about Echinacea and decided to buy some for him, starting with four doses a day. James noticed an immediate physical difference: the tingling James experienced felt positive, and he started to feel stronger and more energized. He also felt better emotionally, and his depression started to lift.

Growing, harvesting, and processing

ALTHOUGH THE ROOT *is the main part of the plant used for medicinal purposes, some herbal manufacturers add a proportion of leaf and seed in their composite tincture. This is a useful option when growing your own plants and making your own tinctures.*

ABOVE **The root is the main part of the plant used in herbal remedies.**

GROWING ECHINACEA

Echinacea can be grown from both seeds and seedlings. The easiest and most successful method, however, is to obtain small plants and transplant them into rich, well-drained soil, mulched with compost.

Planting and germination

Echinacea purpurea is the easiest species to grow at home, and thrives in both full sun and shaded areas. It survives well in most climates, except in consistently very hot and dry

ABOVE **Leaves are harvested in the late spring before the buds have appeared.**

conditions when it should be placed in partial shade. Plant the seeds in the early winter or, if you're using seedlings, transplant them in the early spring.

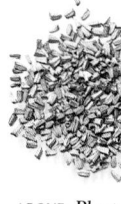

ABOVE **Plants can be grown from seed, though seedlings are more reliable.**

The soil should be well-drained, with a pH of 5.5–6. This species grows particularly well in sandy, fine silt-loam soil, particularly if the soil contains lime.

E. angustifolia and E. pallida are very drought resistant and can survive

SCIENTIFIC TESTING FOR READINESS

Analysis of plant chemistry levels using chromatography gives a scientific viewpoint for optimum harvesting time. There are no standardized criteria as yet, but some herb farms in several countries do test before harvesting. This can include the water content in the root (which should not be more than 10%) and the ash content (no more than 9%).

through the summer with very little water. *E. angustifolia*, in particular, does not grow successfully if the soil is consistently saturated. If possible, use a moderately coarse textured soil (sandy loam), consisting of lime and gravel, to encourage drainage. The soil pH should be 6–8.

BELOW *Leaf growth is vigorous in the spring, before flowers appear.*

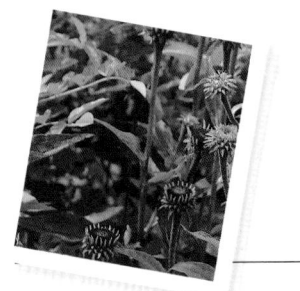

E. angustifolia and *E. pallida* often require a cold, light environment to encourage germination. If you experience any problems, put an overripe banana near the seeds: this will release ethylene gas, a natural growth hormone, and will stimulate germination.

HARVESTING

Commercial In Germany the roots are sometimes harvested in April, before the leaves produce much growth, but in the United States they are more frequently harvested in the fall. The idea is to harvest the root at a time when the plant has died back, so that the energy and plant chemistry is maximized in the root. The root is harvested by cutting the top off the whole plant, leaving about 2in (5cm) of the plant above ground level. A digger then lifts the plant, cutting down to a depth of 12in (30cm).

The leaves are harvested in the late spring, when maximum young foliage has been produced,

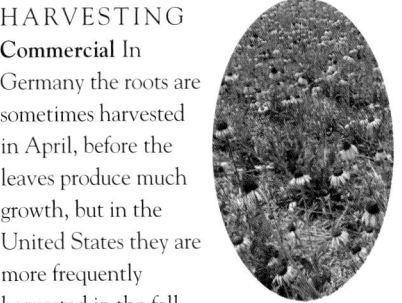

ABOVE *Seeds are harvested at full maturity.*

but before the buds and flowers have appeared. The leaves are harvested by cutting off the tops, leaving 4in (10cm) of the plant above ground level. The harvestable amount of leaves will be greater in the second year than in the first.

Seeds are harvested at full maturity – that is any time in the late summer or in the fall, depending on the climate. Seed heads are usually collected by hand because the delicate central cone can break easily and the seeds scatter.

Homegrown Dig up the roots in the fall, when the chemical constituents are at a premium. Taste the roots: if they produce a strong, tingling numbness in the

mouth, they are ready. The same applies to leaves or seeds: try the leaves for taste when they're young and juicy, well before flowering stalks begin to grow.

When harvesting the leaves, apply the same rules as those used in a commercial harvest: collect them in the late spring, when the leaves are at their most plentiful, but before the buds and flowers appear.

The seeds are ready to be harvested when they are loose enough to come away easily in your hand; they'll not only be at their peak medicinally but will also be capable of germination if you wish.

PROCESSING

Commercial The collected roots are thoroughly washed, dried, and packed. Washing is easy with the long, tap-rooted *E. angustifolia*, but for the fibrous *E. purpurea* it is much harder, at least on a commercial scale, and it helps enormously if the soil is friable and falls away easily.

The roots are then washed with water: when they are scrupulously clean, they are dried at 105–113°F (40–45°C)

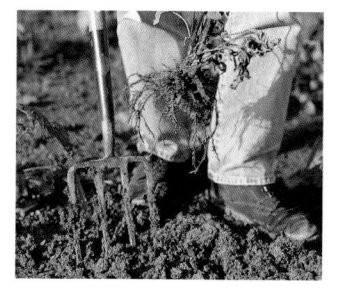

ABOVE *Roots that are to be used should be dug up in the fall after the flowers have seeded.*

until they are brittle. They are graded for quality and then stored on dry, temperature-controlled slatted shelves, or packed in plastic, open-weave sacks, ready for sale.

Leaves are similarly dried, but for a shorter time, and they are stored at lower temperatures.

The complete seed heads are rubbed between boards in order to crush and yield the seeds, and to ensure that the cones and bracts fall away. Finally, the seeds are graded and sold by size and quality.

Homegrown After washing the harvested roots, pat them dry and lay them on cake racks in a warm, dry place.

Alternatively, place the roots on the racks and put them into an oven preheated to 210°F (100°C) but with the heat turned off and the door left open. Cut

very thick roots into smaller pieces to ensure thorough drying.

After collecting the leaves and seeds, put them in brown paper bags and hang them in a very dry place. Every few days take them down and shake them in order to "turn" the contents for better aeration.

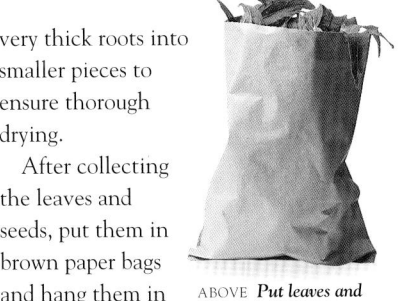

ABOVE *Put leaves and seeds in a paper bag; hang it somewhere dry.*

Once the leaves and seeds feel dry enough, place them in a glass jar. Put on the lid and leave the jar in the sunshine: if water droplets appear, then there is still a moisture content and therefore a risk of spoilage, so you should dry the leaves and seeds further before storing. Store the dried herb, whole or sliced, in airtight containers in a cool, dark place.

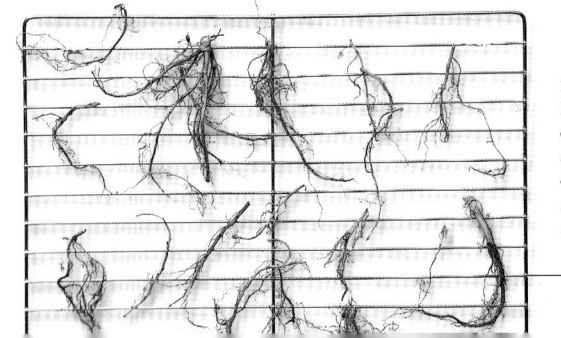

LEFT *Leave harvested roots well spaced on a cake rack in a warm, dry place so that they can dry out.*

Preparations for internal use

THE LEAST COMPLICATED WAY *to take Echinacea is simply to chew the fresh or dried root, leaves, flowers, or seeds. There are, however, more palatable ways to absorb the herb's healing properties.*

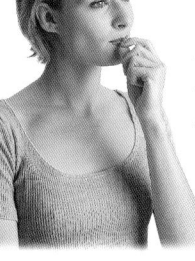

LEFT **The simplest way to take Echinacea is to chew it, as the Native Americans did.**

ECHINACEA ROOT TINCTURE

In this form the herb is concentrated and needs no further preparation for use – and, like capsules and pills, it can be carried around very easily. Echinacea tinctures last a very long time. Some 100-year-old tinctures were found recently and tasted, and the quality appeared not to have suffered at all. However, the herbalist and botanist Christopher Hobbs suggests that a reasonable shelf life for the majority of Echinacea tinctures is two to three years.

You can make a tincture by soaking chopped or shredded roots first in alcohol (to kill any pathogens such as unfriendly bacteria – this is especially important when using fresh herbs) and then in a mixture of alcohol and water. The healing properties of Echinacea are particularly well extracted by water, and the water/alcohol mixture is also important because the polysaccharides in the herb that stimulate the body's immune system don't survive in high concentrations of alcohol.

LEFT **When making a tincture, first soak the chopped roots in alcohol.**

TO MAKE A ROOT TINCTURE

STANDARD QUANTITY

Use 4oz (115g) of dried root or 8oz (225g)
of fresh, with enough vodka to cover – minimum 2 cups (450ml)

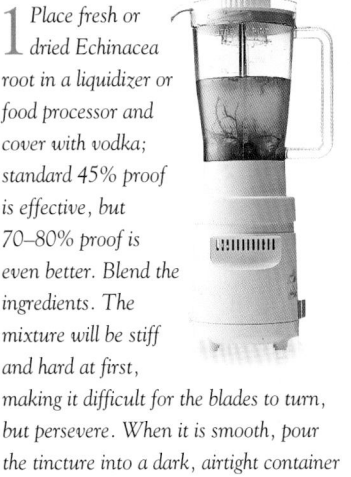

1 *Place fresh or dried Echinacea root in a liquidizer or food processor and cover with vodka; standard 45% proof is effective, but 70–80% proof is even better. Blend the ingredients. The mixture will be stiff and hard at first, making it difficult for the blades to turn, but persevere. When it is smooth, pour the tincture into a dark, airtight container – a dark glass jar or Mason jar is ideal.*

2 *Shake well, label your jar carefully, then store it in a cool place, out of direct sunlight.*

3 *After two days, measure the contents and add water. For dried roots the amount of water is 20% of the volume of vodka if using 45% proof vodka, and 50–60% more water if using 70–80% proof vodka. For fresh roots, add half the amount of water, irrespective of vodka strength used. Leave the jar for 2–4 weeks.*

4 *Strain through a jelly bag, preferably overnight, until you have the last drop. For best results, use a wine press.*

5 *Pour the liquid into dark jars; label and store in a cool, dark place. For personal use, decant into a 2fl oz (50ml) tincture bottle. For dosages, see page 32.*

TINCTURES AND THE MOON'S PHASES

Herbalists occasionally time the production of tinctures to coincide with the gravitational waxing and waning of the moon. To do this, start the process when the moon is new, then strain and bottle at the full moon.

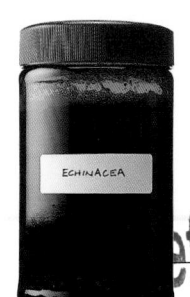

ECHINACEA

TINCTURE FROM LEAVES OR SEEDS

A tincture can be made from Echinacea leaves or seeds as well as the roots – or a mixture of all three. Use the same quantities of liquids as for the roots. Clean utensils in boiling water: for best results add 1–2 drops of essential oil, such as thyme, lavender, or tea tree, to the cleaning water.

REMOVING THE ALCOHOL

You may wish to avoid the small amount of alcohol in the tincture, especially if you're diabetic or if you're expecting a baby. In this case, add a little boiling water to your dose and let it stand for five minutes: roughly 98.5% of the alcohol will evaporate. To avoid alcohol completely, substitute the same quantity of apple cider vinegar for the vodka.

LEFT *For those wishing to avoid alcohol, use apple cider vinegar instead of vodka.*

RECOMMENDED DOSAGES FOR TINCTURES FROM ROOTS, LEAVES, AND SEEDS

🌿 **Everyday use** *Take 1 tsp (5ml) of tincture diluted in 5 tsp (25ml) of water (not fruit juice), 2–3 times daily.*

🌿 **Acute conditions** *Increase the dose frequency to every ½ hour until severe symptoms subside.*

🌿 **Long term** *Take 1 tsp (5ml) of tincture diluted in about 5 tsp (25ml) of water, 2–3 times daily. Repeat this for 10 days on and 4 days off over a period of 1–2 months. With professional guidance, this treatment can be prolonged over a further period.*

ABOVE *Make a tincture from roots, leaves, or seeds to preserve Echinacea's healing qualities.*

🌿 **Children aged 7–12 years** *Take one half of the adult dose in each case for each of the above.*

🌿 **Children aged 3–7 years** *Take one quarter of the adult dose in each case for each of the above.*

🌿 **Children aged below 3 years** *Take two to five drops twice daily.*

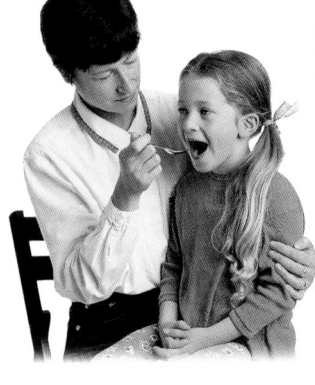

LEFT **A sweet
tincture syrup will
appeal to children.**

CASE STUDY: TONSILS

Jane was troubled by persistently swollen glands and enlarged tonsils. She always felt run down and lacking in energy. At the suggestion of a friend, she took 1 teaspoon (5ml) of Echinacea tincture 3 times a day. She started to feel stronger with each intake, so within a day or two she upped the dose to 1 teaspoon hourly for a few days. She continued to feel better, and the experience also provided her with the springboard for a renewed life based on taking other herbs and making various dietary changes.

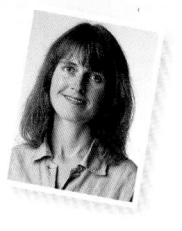

ECHINACEA TINCTURE SYRUP

Most children like the herb's tingling effects, but for those who prefer the taste of something sweeter, try making this tincture syrup.

TO MAKE TINCTURE SYRUP

STANDARD QUANTITY

The quantity of herb tincture used is a matter of choice; and it can be made from roots, leaves, and seeds. The key element is the proportion of added honey.

1 *Mix together 50–80% tincture and 20–50% cold-pressed, organic, runny honey.*

2 *Put the mixture in a glass jar. Shake well before each dose. To make the syrup even tastier, give it a minty flavor by adding* *half a drop of peppermint essential oil to each 2 cups (475ml) of the tincture syrup.*

Recommended dosage

🌿 *Take as for tincture from roots, leaves, and seeds (see opposite).*

ECHINACEA DECOCTION

Water-based processes preserve all the qualities of Echinacea very efficiently. Decoction is therefore a good way to prepare the roots and seeds. Dried roots and seeds may be used, although fresh is always best.

DECOCTION SYRUP

A decoction syrup is made in the same way as the tincture syrup, but uses a decoction as its base instead of a tincture. Take the same dose as for a decoction, adding honey to taste, but do not add the peppermint oil.

TO MAKE A DECOCTION

STANDARD QUANTITY

¾oz (20g) of dried or 1½oz (40g) of fresh roots and/or seeds to 3 cups (700ml) of cold water, reduced to about 2 cups (500ml) of liquid after simmering.

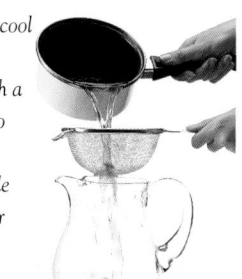

1 *Put the roots and/or seeds in a saucepan (a double boiler is ideal) with the water. Initially boil for 1 minute, then simmer on a very low heat for 20–30 minutes. During this time the liquid should reduce by a third.*

2 *Leave to cool and then strain through a sieve and into a pitcher, keeping a little aside for your* first cup. *Put the pitcher in a cool place. If storing for longer than a day, put it in the refrigerator; it will keep for 3 days. If time is limited strain off the mixture while it is still hot, straight into a thermos. Have a cup immediately, then drink the rest from the thermos.*

Recommended dosage

Adults: 3–4 cups daily. Halve the amount for children aged 7–12, quarter it for those aged 3–7, and a few sips at a time, totaling 6 tsp (30ml) a day, for those under 3.

ECHINACEA INFUSION

Teas are usually made from the delicate parts of a plant that grow above ground. In the case of Echinacea, the leaves, flowers, or even the seeds are used. With both the infusion and the decoction, adults should aim to consume 2 cups (500ml) per day.

ECHINACEA TEA

If you haven't got a tea sock, this tea can also be made in a special teapot infuser, or in a coffee pot with a plunger.

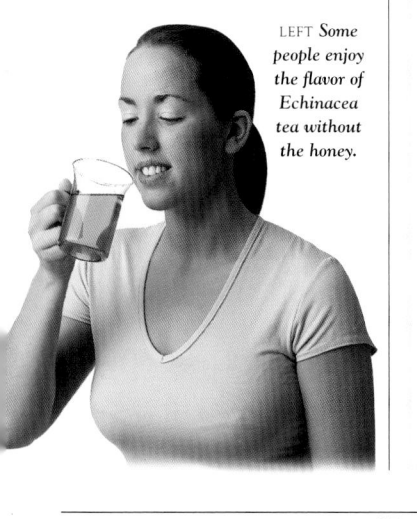

LEFT **Some people enjoy the flavor of Echinacea tea without the honey.**

TO MAKE AN INFUSION

STANDARD QUANTITY

1 tsp (2–3g) of dried or 2 tsp (4–6g) of fresh herb to 1 cup (250ml) of water
OR
⅔oz (20g) of dried herb or 1¼oz (35g) of fresh herb to 2 cups (500ml) of water.

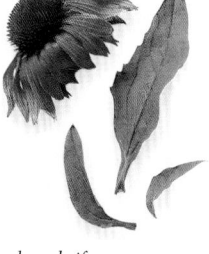
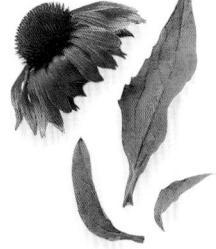

1 *Put the herb in a tea sock and place in a cup or teapot. Pour on boiling water and let it stand for 7–10 minutes.*

2 *Remove the tea sock and, if desired, add ½ tsp (2.5ml) organic, cold-pressed honey to sweeten. However, it's worth noting that teas are usually best drunk without added sweetness and that Echinacea has a very interesting flavor of its own.*

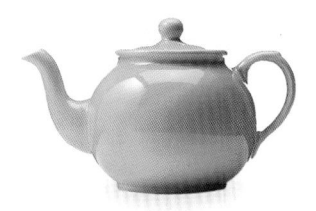

Recommended dosage
Adults and children should take the same dose as for a decoction (see opposite).

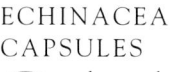
ECHINACEA CAPSULES

Capsules can be made from the dried, powdered root of the herb, not the fresh herb. Freeze-dried powdered root in capsules can also be bought commercially. Capsules make an ideal "portable" remedy.

RIGHT **It is quite easy to make your own capsules from the powdered herb.**

CASE STUDY: ENERGY

Joanne was a 25-year-old schoolteacher who had recently married and bought an old house. She and her husband started to do the house up, but she found that she kept suffering from sore throats and was starting to feel tired and low. She took Echinacea tincture four times a day for two days and found that her sore throat, which usually lasted a week, disappeared much sooner. After that Joanne took Echinacea whenever she felt a sore throat coming on. Over time her energy levels rose, her immune system strengthened, and the sore throat episodes decreased dramatically.

TO MAKE CAPSULES

STANDARD QUANTITY

Approximately 250–300mg of powdered herb fits into a size 00 capsule. Gelatin-free capsules for vegetarians are also available.

1 *Put a little dried, finely powdered Echinacea in a saucer and open up the capsule.*

2 *Using the capsule ends as shovels, push them together until each end is full (one end will be less so), then slide the capsule ends together carefully.*

Recommended dosage
Adults: 2 capsules 2–4 times daily. Children: aged 7–12, 1 capsule 2–4 times daily; aged 3–7, 1 capsule twice daily.

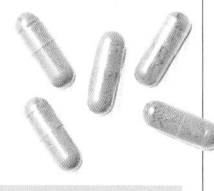

BELOW **Use the ends of the capsule to fill each other.**

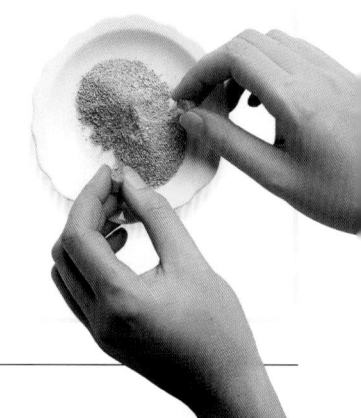

SUGGESTED DOSAGES

DOSE/CONDITION	DURATION	TINCTURE	CAPSULE	TABLET
Acute dose for ailments such as colds and infections	10 days	1 tsp (5ml) 4 times daily or every ½–1 hour	3–4 capsules every 2 hours	1–2 tablets every 2 hours
Maintenance dose after acute stage above, or to prevent disease	2 months	½ tsp (2.5ml) twice daily	2 capsules twice daily	1 tablet twice daily
Chronic, deep-seated conditions such as postviral fatigue syndrome	3–4 months with 4-day breaks every 10 days	2 tsp (10ml) twice daily	6 capsules 4 times daily	4 tablets 4 times daily
Children's dose	As appropriate to situation, but consult a herbalist if in doubt	After breast-feeding and up to 3 years: 2–5 drops daily 3–6 years: 10 drops daily 7–10 years: 20 drops once or twice daily 10–12 years: 30 drops once or twice daily Over 12 years: adult dose Note: Drops give greater accuracy than teaspoons for children's doses, but measure them out beforehand.		

CAUTION

These doses are given only as a guide. Do not exceed the quantities given, or the length of time for treatment. Always consult an accredited herbalist before using Echinacea, or any other herbal remedy, if you are suffering from any serious illness such as cancer.

ABOVE **Herbal remedies should be stored in dark glass bottles or jars.**

Preparations for external use

ECHINACEA IS AN INVALUABLE AID *against a wide range of external conditions as well as internal complaints. It is very effective applied as an ointment, in baths, as dusting powder, and in compresses.*

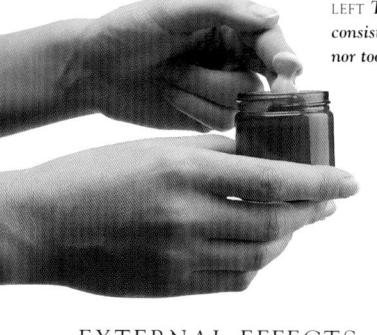

LEFT *The ointment is the right consistency when it is neither too hard nor too runny to stick to the fingers.*

ECHINACEA OINTMENT

Echinacea ointment is useful for treating bites, cuts, wounds, dry eczema, and psoriasis. However, it is *not* appropriate for inflamed, wet, or oozing skin conditions. In these cases, a cooling Echinacea infusion or powdered Echinacea applied to the skin would be much more appropriate.

EXTERNAL EFFECTS OF ECHINACEA

Echinacea is especially effective against a variety of skin conditions and wounds. Its powerful chemistry goes to work immediately at the site of the problem, quickly activating the immune system, where it is most needed. It is a good idea to take the herb internally as well (see pages 30–37), in order to reinforce general immunity.

ECHINACEA BATH

To help treat severe skin problems such as psoriasis or a chickenpox rash, try adding 2 cups (500ml) Echinacea decoction to a shallow bath. The bathwater temperature can be warm or cool.

TO MAKE AN OINTMENT

STANDARD QUANTITY

A good standard is 1½ cups (350ml) of olive oil to 11oz (325g) of dried, not fresh, herbs.

1 Pour the olive oil onto the powdered herbs. Put the mixture in a closed container (ovenproof if you are using the oven method – choose stainless steel, earthenware, unchipped enamel, or ovenproof glass).

2 Put the container into an oven preheated to 100°F (38°C) and heat for an hour, or stand it in the sun or some other warm spot for a week. Stir periodically with a fork.

3 If using the oven method, leave for a further week to macerate, and then heat up again for an hour at the same temperature before straining off. Strain the mixture by passing it through a colander lined with muslin, or by using a jelly bag and hanging it up overnight.

4 Melt 1¾oz (50g) of beeswax in a double boiler or thick-based saucepan at a very low temperature. Mix in the herbal olive oil mixture. Check a little of the mixture for consistency: it is ready for use when it sticks to your fingers without being too hard or too runny. Put it into dark glass jars, then label the jars clearly.

BELOW **Strain the mixture through a colander lined with muslin.**

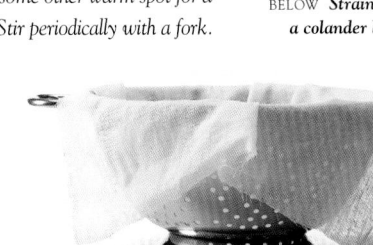

ECHINACEA COMPRESS

For a compress, you will need to make up an Echinacea decoction (see page 34). The decoction can be used either cold or warm. Dip a soft cloth into it, wring it out, and apply it to the affected area. Use cold liquid to ease hot, dry skin conditions, and hot liquid to treat cold, wet skin conditions.

CASE STUDY: RHINITIS

Lily was an energetic mother in her thirties with a parttime job as a careers advisor. She suffered from rhinitis – a recurrent runny nose often caused by an allergy – which plagued her at monthly intervals.

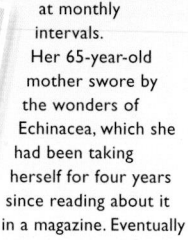

Her 65-year-old mother swore by the wonders of Echinacea, which she had been taking herself for four years since reading about it in a magazine. Eventually Lily decided to give it a try. She took it regularly for two weeks and then stopped. Her rhinitis was late in appearing, and when she got the first symptoms she took the Echinacea again for just one evening. The following morning the anticipated bout of rhinitis failed to appear.

TO MAKE A COMPRESS

STANDARD QUANTITY

Use 3–4 cups of prepared decoction (see page 34)

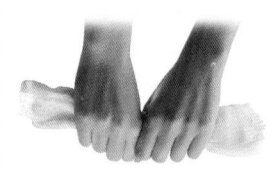

1 *Soak a soft, clean cloth (cheesecloth is ideal) in the decoction and then wring out the excess. Place the compress on the affected area and secure firmly with a bandage held in place by safety pins, or wrap the compress in plastic wrap, which should adhere to itself.*

2 *Leave for 10–20 minutes and then repeat. You can reapply the compress two or three times, leaving the last one on for about 1–2 hours.*

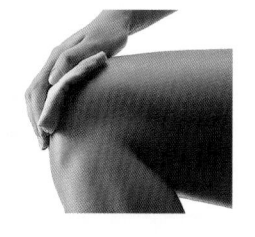

OTHER APPLICATIONS

Gargle

Gargle with Echinacea tea or decoction if you have a tooth abscess or gingivitis. This can be done several times a day. Spit out the liquid after gargling – do not swallow – in case there is pus or toxic debris in the mouth. Echinacea makes a good mouthwash and gargle for other oral infections, such as sore throats, tonsillitis, mouth ulcers, and gum infections.

Cleansing wash

Use Echinacea tea as a wash for infected wounds and rashes, pimples, and pus-filled spots.

Eye bath

Use cooled Echinacea tea to fill an eye bath and rinse the eyes once a day for 3 days, or once a day two or three times a week. If you are eye rinsing for a long period, say 7 days or more, add a few grains of salt to the tea to offset salt and mineral loss from the eye. You can use any salt, but if you decide to use coarse salt, it is important to ensure the grains are fully dissolved in the tea.

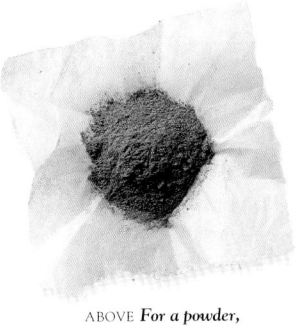

ABOVE *For a powder, sieve commercially produced powdered root.*

Dusting powder

Sieve powdered Echinacea root until it is very fine. This is useful for dusting onto wet psoriasis, eczema, and deep, fleshy wounds.

Juice

Juice pressed from the fresh root is a delightful as well as extremely powerful form of Echinacea. You will need a vegetable/fruit extractor, not the liquidizer used for the tincture. A little goes a long way: 5 tsp (25ml) 3 times daily is ideal for adults, though use up to 7 tsp (35ml) if necessary. For children aged 3–11, use 3 tsp (15ml) spread through the day; 2 tsp (10ml) through the day for toddlers up to 3 years; and 1 tsp (5ml) through the day for babies.

Natural medicine for everyone

ECHINACEA IS BELIEVED to be safe even for those people considered to be especially vulnerable – pregnant and breast-feeding women, children, and the elderly.

PREGNANCY

According to *Herbology throughout the Reproductive Cycle* (American College of Nurse-Midwives, 1994), Echinacea is safe for people of all ages and may be used in moderation during pregnancy. It suggests that "As with most anti-microbials, it is probably wise not to use Echinacea for months at a time, but rather during times of illness or exposure to sickness."

Since pregnant women are advised not to use antibiotics, Echinacea is an excellent alternative and

RIGHT *Guidelines for breast-feeding when using Echinacea are much the same as for pregnancy.*

will help both mother and baby to flourish. It can help minimize or shorten many illnesses.

CHILDREN

It's quite safe for children of all ages to use Echinacea, provided you don't mix it with fruit juice (see page 21). Using a dropper bottle, you can give any liquid form of Echinacea, a few drops at a time, to a baby or toddler who is no longer being breast-fed. To treat a baby that is being breast-fed, the mother should take the Echinacea.

Tinctures (with added liquid organic honey), decoctions (sweetened in a similar way), or premade syrups are also fine. Giving Echinacea to children instead of routinely prescribed antibiotics will greatly enhance the child's immune system – not only in the short term but also for life. This is because the body will be left to fight its own battles, giving the immune system the chance to recognize invading cells and strengthen its own fighting response. However, some serious illnesses may still require antibiotics, so when in doubt, consult your doctor.

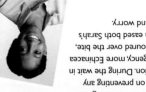

ABOVE *Honey can safely be added to the tincture for children.*

ELDERLY PEOPLE

I t is also safe for older people to take Echinacea. It is a wonderful herb to have at hand for use as needed, particularly because the immune system often weakens during the aging process.

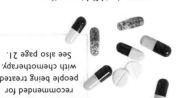

ABOVE *Echinacea is a great benefit to people whose immune systems are weakened by age.*

CASE STUDY: A BAD BITE

Fifteen-year-old Sarah loved dogs, but when she patted a strange dog in the street one day, it responded with a vicious bite. Her mother always had Echinacea at home and doused the wound in liberal amounts of the tincture. It stung but went straight to work on preventing any infection. During the wait in emergency, more Echinacea was poured over the bite, which eased both Sarah's pain and worry.

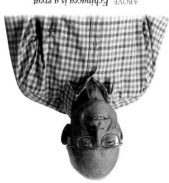

ABOVE *Avoid Echinacea if you are on drugs that suppress the function of the immune system.*

Herbal combinations

HERBAL COMBINATIONS CAN be used when the effect of a single herb needs complementing in a certain way, but if you are pregnant, breastfeeding or have a serious medical condition, consult your doctor or qualified herbalist first.

Many herbal formulas consist of one main herb with one or two others to support it. Other formulas have one principal herb, with many other herbs working to assist or create a "rainbow effect." The main herb may be required to soothe impaired tissue, while the rest are there to nourish, to help eliminate toxins, and to assist in nerve and blood supply.

Some formulas have equal quantities of four or five herbs, their similar actions working in slightly different ways.

LEFT *Herbal formulas may contain many different herbs.*

POSTVIRAL FATIGUE SYNDROME (ME)

This formula helps to treat ME by boosting immunity levels.

Formula 3 parts Echinacea root, 3 parts Burdock root, 3 parts Pau d'arco inner bark, 2 parts Garlic cloves, and ¼ part Cayenne pods.

Dosage Adult: 1 tsp (5ml) of tincture formula 3 or 4 times daily. Children aged 7–12: half adult dose.

Pau d'arco metabolizes oxygen and is a powerful immune system supporter, useful for treating postviral fatigue syndrome.

Garlic supports the immune system, while Cayenne helps to provide a good blood supply and replenishes oxygen.

Burdock boosts the immune system and cleanses the blood.

THRUSH

This condition is a fungal overgrowth caused by the organism *Candida albicans*. It thrives in the presence of alcohol, so this formula is best made up as a decoction.

Formula equal parts Echinacea root, Pau d'arco inner bark, and Burdock root.

Dosage 3 cups (500ml) daily as a decoction, or 1 tsp (5ml) 3 or 4 times daily as an alcohol-free tincture (see page 32).

All three herbs are highly stimulating to the immune system, particularly against all types of fungi. Echinacea helps the destruction of dying off yeasts, and the Burdock root will act as a blood cleanser,

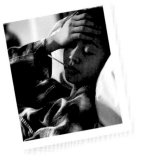

RIGHT *The early symptoms of the common cold can be eased using Echinacea root.*

ABOVE **Pau d'arco inner bark boosts the immune system.**

diuretic, and pancreatic balancer (pancreatic imbalance is often a contributory factor to the original problem).

Pau d'arco inner bark is an all-round immune booster, and works particularly well against chronic fungal conditions; it also supports the pancreas and, like Echinacea, is anti-inflammatory.

COLDS AND FLU

This formula is best taken as a tincture or tea at a disease's onset. It combines Echinacea with cold and flu herbs such as Peppermint leaves, Yarrow leaves, and Elderflower, which stimulate sweating and dry out mucous membranes.

Formula 3 parts Echinacea root, 1 part Peppermint leaves, with a dash of Cayenne (or a few Cayenne pods).

Dosage 1 tsp (5ml) 5 times daily OR

Formula 4 parts Echinacea root, 2 parts Yarrow leaves, 1 part Elderflower, and 1 part Peppermint leaves.

Dosage Adults: 1 tsp (5ml) of tincture formula every 2 hours. Children: aged 7–12, half adult dose; aged 3–7, quarter adult dose; under 3 years, 3 drops every 2 hours.

COUGHS, BRONCHIAL AND UPPER RESPIRATORY INFECTIONS

The following herbs would be ideal made up as a tincture, with some elderberry syrup added to give the formula an all-round soothing effect.

Formula 2 parts Echinacea root, 2 parts Elecampane root, and 2 parts Elderberry syrup.

To make Elderberry syrup, half fill a large jar or Mason jar with elderberries, and cover with vegetable glycerine. Purée in a blender, then return to the jar and top up with spring water. Shake well, cover, and let stand in a sunny spot for 2 weeks. Shake the jar daily. After 2 weeks sieve the berries and return to a clean jar.

Dosage Adults: 1 tsp (5ml) 3 or 4 times daily. Children: aged 7–12, half adult dose; aged 3–7, quarter adult dose; under 3 years, 3 drops 3 or 4 times daily.

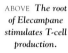

ABOVE *The root of Elecampane stimulates T-cell production.*

Like the roots of Echinacea and Burdock, Elecampane contains inulin. This increases the production of T-cells and the activity of other killer cells that destroy virus-infected cells – it is a specific remedy for respiratory disorders.

Elderberry is antiviral and is rich in vitamin C.

Echinacea eases inflamed lungs and stimulates the immune system.

LOW METABOLISM AND WEAKNESS

Echinacea will help stimulate an immune response in people with low metabolisms who are inclined to feel cold, have low body weight, and poor powers of recovery. However, if Echinacea is not supported by other good tonics, full recovery will be difficult. The problem may drag on or, in some cases, may get worse. This can happen with a very persistent cough, for instance. If weight loss and other signs of deficiency have set in, seek qualified medical help immediately.

> **CAUTION**
>
> Do not use Elecampane if you are pregnant: make the remedy using only the other herbs.

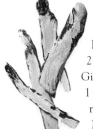

ABOVE *Astragalus root gently helps the body deal with stress.*

Formula 3 parts Echinacea root, 2 parts Siberian Ginseng root, 1 part Astragalus root, and ½ part Marshmallow root.

Dosage Adults: 1 tsp (5ml) of tincture formula 3–5 times daily. Children: aged 7–12, half adult dose; aged 3–7, quarter adult dose; under 3 years, 3 drops 3 or 4 times daily.

Siberian Ginseng root is capable of creating a highly beneficial balanced support to the body and has no side effects. While it helps to boost energy, it never overstimulates – it simply helps the body adapt to stresses. Astragalus works in a very similar way.

Marshmallow root provides a good tonic for the whole body and is a specific remedy for debilitating conditions that make patients feel low.

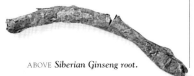

ABOVE *Siberian Ginseng root.*

SKIN CONDITIONS

Herbs that treat psoriasis, eczema, and other inflammatory skin conditions should also enhance the general detoxification of the body, especially the liver. This formula aims to support the digestive tract and immune system, and clear the lymph system and bloodstream. It also helps to clear and "cool" the liver, and aids the kidneys and bowel to excrete the collected toxins and debris from the body.

> **CAUTION**
>
> Do not use Echinacea if there are any signs of adrenal exhaustion in autoimmune diseases or cancers, where levels of white blood cells are excessive.

Formula 2 parts Echinacea root, 1 part Barberry root bark, 1 part Turmeric rhizome, 1 part Cleavers herb, 1 part Dandelion root.

Dosage Same dosage as for coughs (see opposite).

Echinacea helps to treat many skin complaints, including those linked to impaired digestion, a sluggish or "hot" liver, and the presence of inflammation and opportunistic pathogens such as unfriendly bacteria and fungi.

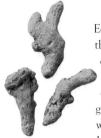

ABOVE *Turmeric rhizome is anti-inflammatory*

Barberry will support Echinacea's work on the liver, dredging and drawing it, helping it to function more efficiently, and getting the bowel to work smoothly. However, before taking Barberry, pregnant women should consult a qualified herbalist.

Like Echinacea, Turmeric is anti-inflammatory, with an action even stronger than hydrocortisone (a steroid hormone used to treat inflammation and allergies). It assists the liver by increasing bile flow and has a protective action on both the liver and the stomach. This ancient herb is used in Chinese and Ayurvedic medicine as a digestive aid and blood cleanser (see pages 22-3).

Cleavers herb is a general detoxifier and lymph cleanser and, with the Dandelion root, will safely clear the kidneys.

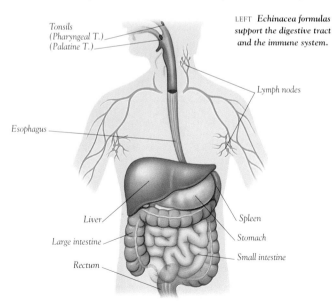

LEFT *Echinacea formulas support the digestive tract and the immune system.*

Tonsils
(Pharyngeal T.)
(Palatine T.)

Lymph nodes

Esophagus

Liver

Spleen

Large intestine

Stomach

Rectum

Small intestine

TONSILLITIS

This combination of herbs will make a tincture to help ease tonsil inflammation.

Formula 2 parts Echinacea root, 2 parts Elderberry syrup (see page 46), 1 part Poke root, ⅛ part Cayenne pod.

Dosage 1 tsp (5ml) 4 or 5 times daily until 3 days after symptoms have eased. Dose can be increased to every half hour while pain is acute, but for no longer than 2 days without medical advice.

Echinacea is tailor-made for tonsillitis because of its immediate, slightly numbing action in the mouth and throat. The relief from pain can often last from dose to dose if there is a half hour between them. Echinacea also mobilizes the immune system.

Elderberry soothes the throat and, being antiviral, will also help the immune system.

Poke root is quite a strong herb for this condition, but it is good to use for a limited period of time – 3 weeks normally, and not more than 3 months – because it will quickly purify and decongest the bloodstream and lymph system. It also keeps the bowels moving.

URETHRITIS

This painful infection of the urethra, the tube that conducts urine from the bladder to the exterior, affects mainly women. Echinacea, combined with other herbs, will help to combat the cause of the infection.

Formula 2 parts Echinacea root, 1 part Uva Ursi leaves, 1 part Corn Silk, and 1 part Barberry root bark.

Dosage 1 tsp (5ml) of tincture formula 3 or 4 times daily. If acute, a night dose of 1 tsp (5ml) at two separate intervals may also be taken.

Echinacea will mobilize the immune system to fight the microbial infection, whether the cause is bacterial, fungal, or viral.

Uva Ursi is especially useful for the urinary tract, where it will cleanse, disinfect, and heal the affected area.

Corn Silk has similar abilities to Uva Ursi but acts in a slightly varying and complementary way.

Barberry root bark will help to treat the infection if it is of fungal origin, and it will also help to decongest the liver, thereby lightening the load on the whole body.

Conditions chart

THIS CHART *is a guide to some of the ailments that Echinacea can treat, but it is not intended to replace other forms of treatment. Always consult your doctor or another qualified medical practitioner before embarking on a course of treatment.*

NAME	INTERNAL USE	EXTERNAL USE
ACNE	Tincture or capsule, or decoction and tincture	Decoction washed over skin, once daily
ALLERGIES such as urticaria and hay fever	Tincture or capsule, or decoction and tincture	Decoction wash, 2 or 3 times daily
ASTHMA Precipitated by or complicated by infection	Tincture or capsule, or decoction and tincture	
BARBER'S RASH		Ointment daily or decoction wash, daily
BRONCHITIS	Tincture or capsule, or decoction and tincture	
BURNS Use topically unless severe, in which case also take internally	Tincture or capsule, or decoction and tincture	Ointment or decoction wash and/or dusting powder, 1–3 times daily

NAME	INTERNAL USE	EXTERNAL USE
CANDIDA	Tincture or capsule, or decoction and tincture	
COLD SORES	Tincture or capsule, or decoction and tincture	Ointment, hourly at first then 3 times daily
COMMON COLD	Tincture or capsule, or decoction and tincture	
COUGH	Tincture or capsule, or decoction and tincture	
CROUP	Tincture or capsule, or decoction and tincture	
DERMATITIS	Tincture or capsule, or decoction and tincture	Ointment or decoction wash, twice daily
ECZEMA	Tincture or capsule, or decoction and tincture	Ointment or dusting powder or decoction wash, twice daily
ENTERITIS	Tincture or capsule, or decoction and tincture	
FOOD POISONING	Tincture or capsule, or decoction and tincture	

NAME	INTERNAL USE	EXTERNAL USE
FUNGAL INFECTIONS	Tincture or capsule, or decoction and tincture	Ointment or dusting powder or decoction wash, twice daily
GERMAN MEASLES	Tincture or capsule, or decoction and tincture	Ointment or dusting powder or decoction wash, 2–3 times a day up to hourly
INFLUENZA	Tincture or capsule, or decoction and tincture	
INSECT BITES	Tincture or capsule, or decoction and tincture	Tincture at site of puncture, every 5 minutes
MEASLES	Tincture or capsule, or decoction and tincture	Ointment or dusting powder or decoction wash, 2–3 times daily up to hourly
MUMPS	Tincture or capsule, or decoction and tincture	
PSORIASIS	Tincture or capsule, or decoction and tincture	Ointment or dusting powder or decoction wash, 2–3 times daily

NAME	INTERNAL USE	EXTERNAL USE
SHINGLES	Tincture or capsule, or decoction and tincture	Ointment or dusting powder or decoction wash, 2–3 times daily up to hourly
SINUSITIS	Tincture or capsule, or decoction and tincture	
SKIN PROBLEMS	Tincture or infusion or decoction	Ointment, 2–3 times daily
SORE THROAT	Tincture or infusion or decoction	
SUNBURN Use topically unless severe, in which case also take internally	Tincture or capsule, or decoction and tincture	Ointment or decoction wash, 5 times daily
TONSILLITIS	Tincture or capsule, or decoction and tincture	Gargle hourly to begin with, then 4 times daily
URETHRITIS	Tincture or capsule, or decoction and tincture	Decoction wash, twice daily
VAGINITIS	Tincture or capsule, or decoction and tincture	
WHOOPING COUGH	Tincture or capsule, or decoction and tincture	

How Echinacea works

ECHINACEA IS COMPOSED OF *a number of highly effective active ingredients, which work in different ways on the body's systems.*

Echinacea includes the following ingredients:

❊ Echinacoside: a compound with high antimicrobial abilities. Echinacoside is found mainly in *E. angustifolia*. It is the herb's most active ingredient and gives the strong tingling sensation and numbing metallic effect in the mouth.

❊ Polysaccharides (see page 57): one of these, inulin, increases production of T-cells and other natural killer cells that stimulate the immune system.

❊ Betaine HCL: a digestive enzyme that helps to stimulate digestion.

❊ Flavonoids (quercetin and rutocide): these work as antioxidants by neutralizing damaging atoms and reducing the risk of a number of serious diseases. Flavonoids are partly responsible for the efficiency of macrophages – these are scavenger cells that remove bacteria from the blood.

❊ Nutrients, including small amounts of aluminum, calcium, copper, chlorine, iron, magnesium, potassium, vitamins A and E (useful to immunity), and particularly high levels of vitamin C. Other chemical components include:

❊ Alkaloids such as tussilagin, very helpful for throat

RIGHT **Echinacea contains a large number of trace elements that are important in nutrition.**

VARYING INGREDIENTS

Some of the chemical constituents mentioned here are found only in the roots, others in the parts of the plant growing above ground; some are present only when the herb is fresh or dried. Climate and season can also make a huge difference: for example, inulin concentrations are much higher in the fall and winter than in the spring, so it's best to harvest roots during these seasons. On the other hand, the fructose content is higher in the summer and the fall.

disorders, and cynarin, a bitter substance that helps the liver.

❋ Essential oils: caryophylene, vanillin, and humulene, which are anti-bacterial and stimulate the digestion process.

❋ Tannins: these reduce infection by forming a protective "crest".

❋ Proteins, which carry useful steroids and oxygen.

❋ Fatty acids, which are needed to sustain energy levels and act as the body's building blocks.

MAIN EFFECTS

❋ Promotes cellular immunity.

❋ Stimulates levels of properdin, which kills bacteria and viruses.

❋ Eases inflammation.

❋ Stimulates the production of healthy new tissue, internally and externally, and temporarily strengthens the barrier against invasive organisms that break down tissue.

According to herbalist Christopher Hobbs, the Echinacoside content of the herb helps to balance undesirably high amounts of harmful bacteria, fungi, and viruses, and generally increases resistance to infectious diseases.

In 1989, two controlled studies involving 100 flu patients showed that Echinacea shortened the duration of the flu and eased the symptoms. (*Vorberg and Schneider 1989, Dorn 1989, information courtesy of Christopher Hobbs.*)

RESEARCH RESULTS

Most of the research into Echinacea over the last 20 years has focused on the herb's ability to stimulate the immune system, and findings clearly indicate that its activity in the bloodstream has a value in the defense against tumor cells. Studies in humans have shown that Echinacea helps white blood cells to attack foreign microorganisms and toxins in the bloodstream.

Glossary

AERIAL PARTS

Those parts of the plant that grow above the ground – stem, leaves, and flowers.

ALKALOID

One of a group of substances that contain nitrogen. They are produced by plants and can have strong effects on the function of the body. Many alkaloids are important drugs, including morphine, quinine, atropine, and codeine.

ANTI-INFLAMMATORY

Reduces inflammation.

ANTIMICROBIAL

Destroys or inhibits the growth of microorganisms.

ANTIOXIDANTS

Substances found particularly in high-chlorophyll foods that protect the cells from free-radicals (damaging atoms) and reduce the risk of some serious diseases.

AYURVEDIC MEDICINE

Healing system of ancient East India, which is based on constitutional typing into three basic Doshas (or dispositions): Vata (Air), Pitta (Fire), and Kapha (Water).

BETAINE HCL

(Hydrochloric acid): this is a digestive enzyme that helps to stimulate digestion.

BITTER

Flavor that stimulates secretions of saliva and digestive juices.

CHROMATOGRAPHY

Process that separates and identifies the chemical composition of plants by means of a photographic plate. The active principles are represented on the plate by colored bands.

COMPRESS

Cloth soaked in cold or hot herb decoction for application to the skin.

DECOCTION

Method of preserving and preparing herbs in water.

FLAVONOIDS

Compounds that cause yellow light to be reflected in plants, and are responsible for a wide range of actions including reducing inflammation and fighting fungus.

FRIABLE

Soft, light soil that falls easily through your fingers.

INFUSION

A herb tea used for medicinal purposes. It can be drunk either hot or cold.

INTERLEUKIN

Defense enzyme produced by macrophages that "eats" toxins and tumors.

INULIN

Carbohydrate that is filtered from the bloodstream by the kidneys, so it is used to test kidney function. It stimulates the function of the immune system.

LYMPH CLEANSER

Herb able to assist in motivating and cleansing the part of the immune system that produces T-helper and T-suppressor cells, as well as B-cells.

LANCEOLATE

Lance-shaped – as in the leaf shape of E. *angustifolia*.

MACROPHAGES

Large cells that destroy small particles foreign to themselves, such as toxic chemicals and tumor cells. They are the deep cleansers of the immune system.

PATHOGENS

Unfriendly parasitic microorganisms, such as bacteria, that produce disease.

PHAGOCYTES

Immune system cells that destroy unfriendly microorganisms, cellular debris, and chemicals by ingesting ("eating") them.

POLYSACCHARIDES

Large number of sugars linked together where energy is stored in living tissue.

PROPERDIN

Serum protein capable of neutralizing viruses and bacteria.

RHIZOME

Underground stem that stores nutrients; it is similar to a bulb.

ROOT

Part of the plant that grows underground, absorbing water and mineral salts from the soil.

TINCTURE

Plant medicine prepared by soaking herbs in alcohol and water.

TOPICAL

A treatment that is applied to the surface of the body as opposed to being taken internally.

Further reading

AMERICAN HERBALISM, *Michael Tierra* (The Crossing Press, 1992)

BRITISH HERBAL PHARMACOPOEIA 1983 AND 1996 (British Herbal Medical Association, 1996)

THE COMPLETE ILLUSTRATED HOLISTIC HERBAL, *David Hoffmann* (Element Books Limited, 1996)

ECHINACEA: NATURE'S IMMUNE ENHANCER, *Steven Foster* (Healing Arts Press, 1991)

ECHINACEA "THE IMMUNE HERB", *Christopher Hobbs* (Botanica Press, 1990)

ENCYCLOPAEDIA OF HERBS AND HERBALISM, *Malcolm Stuart* (Black Cat, 1987)

ENCYCLOPAEDIA OF HERBS AND THEIR USES, *Deni Bown* (Dorling Kindersley, 1995)

ENCYCLOPAEDIA OF MEDICINAL PLANTS, *Andrew Chevallier* (Dorling Kindersley, 1996)

ESSENTIAL SCIENCE CHEMISTRY, *Freemantle & Tidy* (Oxford University Press, 1983)

FIELD GUIDE TO THE NORTH EASTERN, NORTH CENTRAL, NORTH AMERICAN WILD FLOWERS, *R. Peterson & M. McKenny* (Houghton Mifflin Co., 1968)

FLOWER ESSENCES: AN ILLUSTRATED GUIDE, *Carol Rudd* (Element Books Limited, 1998)

FOUNDATIONS OF HEALTH, *Christopher Hobbs* (Botanica Press, 1992)

HERBAL PHARMACOLOGY, *Christopher Hobbs* (Botanica Press, 1990)

HOW INDIANS USE WILD PLANTS FOR FOOD, MEDICINE & CRAFTS, *F. Densmore* (Dover Publications Limited, 1974)

INCURABLES, *Dr. Christopher* (Christopher Publications, 1977)

INDIAN USES OF NATIVE PLANTS, *Edith Van Allen Murphey* (Meyerbooks, 1990)

MANUAL OF CONVENTIONAL MEDICINE FOR ALTERNATIVE PRACTITIONERS, *S. Gasgoine* (Jigame Press, 1993)

NUTRITIONAL HERBOLOGY, *Mark Pederson* (Wendell W. Whitman Company, 1994)

OUT OF THIS EARTH, *Simon Mills* (Viking, 1991)

SPIRITUAL PROPERTIES OF HERBS, *Gurudas* (Cassandra Press, 1988)

TEXTBOOK OF ADVANCED HERBOLOGY, *Terry Willard* (Wild Rose College of Natural Healing, 1992)

TEXTBOOK OF MODERN HERBOLOGY, *Terry Willard* (Wild Rose College of Natural Healing, 1993)

Useful addresses

ASSOCIATIONS AND SOCIETIES

British Herbal Medicine Association (B.H.M.A.)
Sun House, Church Street, Stroud,
Glos, GL5 1JL, UK
Tel: 011 44 1453-751389
Fax: 011 44 1453-751402
Works with the Medicine Control Agency to promote high standards of quality and safety of herbal medicine

British Herbal Practitioners Association (B.H.P.A)
Midsummer Cottage and Clinic,
Nether-Wescote, Kingham,
Oxon, OX7 6SD, UK
Tel: 011 44 1993 830 419
Fax: 011 44 1993 830 957
Promotes the availability of professional herbal treatment and raises training and practice standards within the profession

Friends of the Earth
26-28 Underwood Street,
London N1 7JQ, UK
Tel: 011 44 171-490 1555
Britain's leading ecological association

Herb Society
Deddington Hill Farm,
Warmington, Banbury,
Oxon OX17 1XB, UK
Tel: 011 44 1295-692000
Fax: 011 44 1295-692004
Educational charity that disseminates information about herbs

SUPPLIERS IN THE UK

Baldwin & Company
171-173 Walworth Road,
London SE17 1RW, UK
Tel: 011 44 171-703 5550
Herbs, storage bottles, jars, containers

Hambleden Herbs
Court Farm, Milverton,
Somerset TA4 1NE UK
Tel: 011 44 1823-401205
Organic herbs by mail order

Herbs, Hands, Healing
The Cabins, Station Warehouse,
Station Road, Fulham Market,
Norfolk IP21 4XE UK
Tel: 011 44 1379-608007
Tel/fax: 011 44 1379-608201
Herbal formulas, organic herbs, and Superfood

SUPPLIERS/SCHOOLS IN THE USA

American Botanical Pharmacy
PO Box 3027, Santa Monica,
California, USA
Tel/fax: 1310 453-1987
Manufacturer and distributor of herbal products; runs training courses

Blessed Herbs
109 Barre Plains Road,
Oakham,
MA 01068, USA
Dried bulk herbs are available by mail order in order to make your own preparations